Brain Training On Mastermind Techniques

Step By Step Guide On How to Become a Mastermind

By: Leighton K. Baines

9781631871672

Brain Training

PUBLISHER'S NOTES

Disclaimer – Speedy Publishing, LLC

This publication is intended to provide helpful and informative material. It is not intended to diagnose, treat, cure, or prevent any health problem or condition, nor is intended to replace the advice of a physician. No action should be taken solely on the contents of this book. Always consult your physician or qualified healthcare professional on any matters regarding your health and before adopting any suggestions in this book or drawing inferences from it.

The author and publisher specifically disclaim all responsibility for any liability, loss or risk, personal or otherwise, which is incurred as a consequence, directly or indirectly, from the use or application of any contents of this book.

Any and all product names referenced within this book are the trademarks of their respective owners. None of these owners have sponsored, authorized, endorsed, or approved this book.

Always read all information provided by the manufacturers' product labels before using their products. The author and publisher are not responsible for claims made by manufacturers.

This book was originally printed before 2014. This is an adapted reprint by Speedy Publishing LLC with newly updated content designed to help readers with much more accurate and timely information and data.

Speedy Publishing, LLC©2014

40 E. Main Street #1156

Newark, Delaware

19711

Contact Us: 1-888-248-4521

Website: http://www.speedypublishing.com

REPRINTED Paperback Edition: ISBN: 9781631871672

Manufactured in the United States of America

Leighton K. Baines

DEDICATION

This book is dedicated to my parents. They have always encouraged me to not be afraid of working for what I want. I was also encouraged to always keep my mind working and not to let my thoughts or educational aspirations become stagnant.

Brain Training

TABLE OF CONTENTS

Publisher's Notes 2

Dedication 3

Introduction 6

Chapter 1- How Does Our Brain Work 8

Chapter 2- The Brain Hemispheres- Left and Right 10

Chapter 3- Types of Intelligence 12

Chapter 4- "Successful" Intelligence 16

Chapter 5- Styles of Learning 19

Chapter 6- Types of Personality 21

Chapter 7- Self-Assessment 23

Chapter 8- How to Sharpen 25

Chapter 9- How to Enhance Creativity 30

Chapter 10- Easy Problem Solving Techniques 33

Chapter 11- Memory Improvement Techniques 36

Chapter 12- Autotelic Thinking 42

Chapter 13- Maintaining Brain Power 45

Chapter 14- What Is Manifestation? 48

Chapter 15- Why People Have Problems Manifesting 51

Chapter 16- Presumptions about Manifestation 53

Leighton K. Baines
Chapter 17- Setting Your Intention- The Importance of It.......... 55

About The Author.. 60

Brain Training
INTRODUCTION

Have you ever been envious of people who seem to have no end of clever ideas, who are able to think quickly in any situation, or who seem to have flawless memories? Could it be that they're just born smarter or quicker than the rest of us? Or are there some secrets that they might know that we don't?

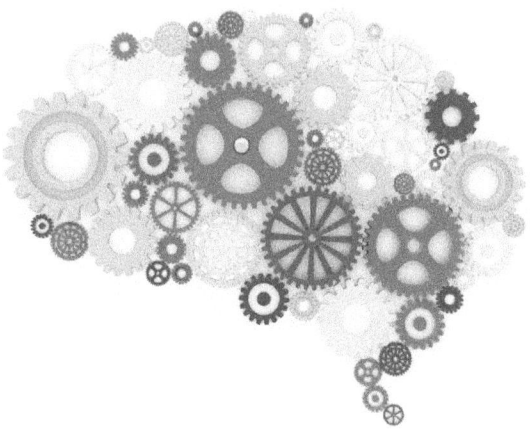

If

- You seem to forget important things
- You have good ideas but they come too late
- You'd like to be better at solving problems
- You wish you could communicate better
- You'd like to be better at tuning out distractions
- You admire creative people and want to be more creative yourself

Leighton K. Baines

- You'd give anything to have a better overall approach to life's challenges,

Then this book is for you. In it you will learn how the brain works in general, the styles related to thinking, your own personal style, and how you might train your brain to think better.

Our brains have vast potential - you may have heard that we only use about 5% of our brains. That's true. But there are techniques we can use to maximize our brain power. By the end of this book, you'll know a lot more about how to maximize your thinking and even your life.

Chapter 1 - How Does Our Brain Work

No doubt about it, our brains are pretty magnificent. Talk about multitasking! We all do it - watch television, read a magazine, realize how great the evening meal smells in the kitchen, listen to the person in the room with us, and be excited about plans for the weekend - all at the same time. We can do this because of our brain's ability to make all kinds of connections.

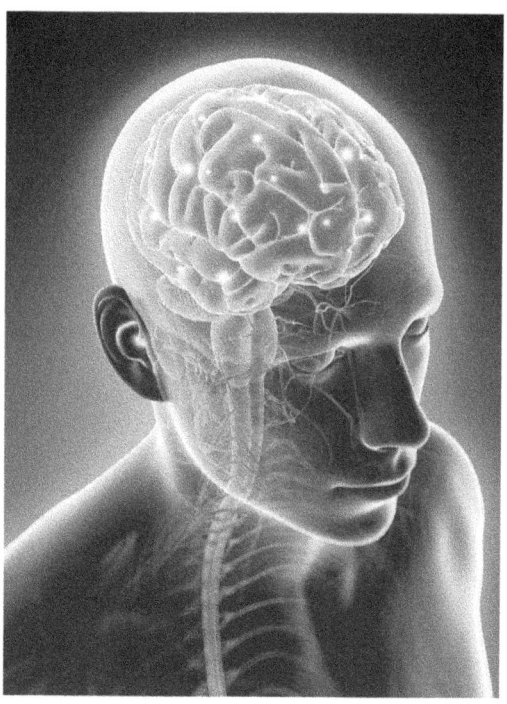

Our brains have developed over thousands of years. Their basic construction can be divided into three parts:

Primitive brain - this region of the brain is about the size of an apricot and controls our basic functions like blood circulation, reading, and indigestion. It also controls our "fight or flight" response to danger, and decides whether we will stay and fight or run away. It's also believed that when we are in stressful situations, the other parts of our brain shut down and leave everything up to the primitive brain, which is why we might find it more difficult to think clearly when we are stressed.

Cerebellum - this part of the brain is called the mammalian brain. It surrounds the primitive brain and processes our emotions and long- term memories. It also processes information learned through our senses.

Cerebral cortex - this covers the primitive brain and the cerebellum and makes up about 80% of our brain area. It determines language, thought, reasoning, complex movement patterns, and other things like appreciation of poetry and music.

In addition to these three parts of the brain, we all have millions of brain cells called neurons. Each neuron has its own special function. Neurons use electrical impulses and chemical reactions to and from the central nervous system and within the brain.

Neurons store information and work together in groups to generate actions and reactions and control specific thoughts. Each neuron has the potential for one million billion connections with other neurons. So, even though we only use 5% of our brain capacity, you can see that there is still an enormous amount of activity in our brains.

Chapter 2 - The Brain Hemispheres - Left and Right

You may have heard the terms left brain and right brain. It wasn't until the 1960s that a scientist named Roger Sperry discovered that different activities are associated with different sides of the brain, thus the term left brain and right brain thinking was coined.

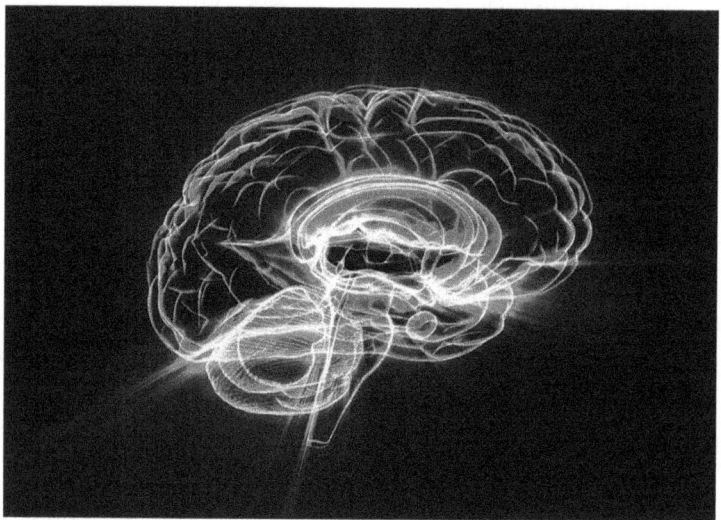

The left side of our brain is the logical side, the mathematical side. It deals with details and organization, and controls our speech and our language. The right side of our brain operates in a less organized way. It handles creativity, interpretation, emotions, imagination, intuition, and spatial awareness.

At one time, scientists thought that these two halves of the brain operated completely independently of each other, but more recent thinking believes that there is some flexibility so that different parts of the brain can learn new functions.

Leighton K. Baines

We all have five senses. Recent evidence shows that the more you are able to use your senses, the better your memory and thinking ability will be. The five senses are sight, hearing, smell, touch, and taste. Our brain interprets the information from the senses to help us act and react and stay out of danger.

It's interesting that, although we all have the same five senses, because of our individual perceptions, we often don't agree on what our senses are telling us. For instance, how many times have you been in a room where it's too hot for you but too cold for someone else? Or vice versa?

How many times have you and someone standing next to you disagreed about what you saw when you were looking at exactly the same thing? How many times have you liked the taste of a new food, but your partner has the opposite reaction? This is all due to our individual perceptions of sensual information.

The brain controls every area of our body. It starts as an electrical burst of activity in the cerebral cortex and moves to the motor cortex, which sends out nerve signals to specific parts of the body. The signals then move down the spinal cord, along the motor nerves, to the muscles.

The signals go to every part of our body and control every action. More complex activities that need body parts with finer control, such as fingers or lips, have bigger areas of the motor cortex.

The brain is beginning to seem like a complicated place, isn't it, but we are just getting started.

Chapter 3 - Types of Intelligence

What Exactly Is IQ?

Many times in the past people were either thought of as intelligent or not intelligent. We've all heard it in school; we've all known who got better grades and who didn't. We all assumed that meant that some people were smarter and some people were not so smart.

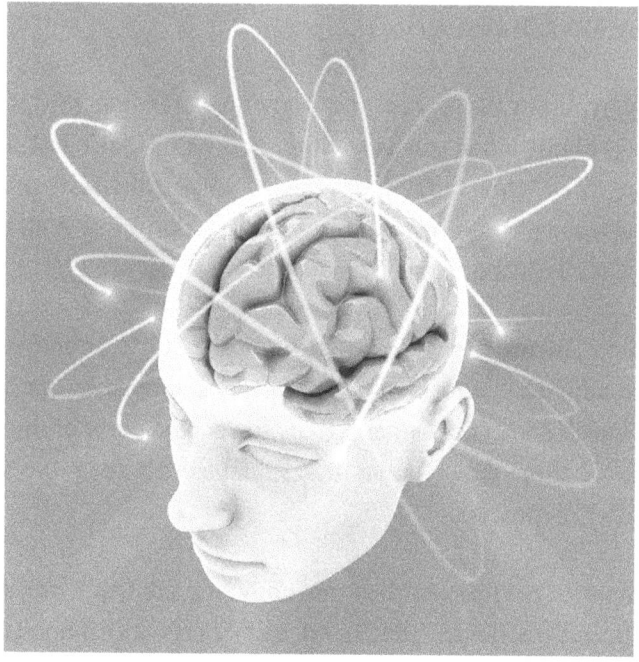

We all probably grew up with intelligence tests, based on language and math, that measured our "intelligence quotient."

These days, we have a broader definition of intelligence. It's no longer limited to being skilled in math and science. It now includes capacity for understanding and describes a person as being intelligent when he can use his mind in a combination of ways.

Scientists are still developing these theories further all time. In fact, all scientists as yet do not agree completely on the terminology. But there's quite a bit of agreement on these ten types of intelligence. We all have more than one of these 10 types; the average is about five.

That accounts for some of us being better at some tasks, and others having mastery over different tasks.

10 Types of Intelligence

Linguistic

People with linguistic intelligence usually have a large vocabulary and often are good at spelling and grammar. These people love stories, languages, and words.

Mathematical

People with mathematical intelligence are good at number puzzles and abstract mathematical problems. They are often good at statistics and notice when statistics are incorrect. They also are usually good at knowing how gadgets work and adept at fixing things.

Visual

If you have visual intelligence, you're likely good and diagrams and illustrations, and you are probably aware of shape, color, and texture. You might understand a new concept more quickly if it's presented with a picture or a diagram. And you might like to doodle.

Physical

Brain Training

This might surprise you, but physical is now considered a type of intelligence. This person enjoys physical activity and is often good at sports or dancing or both. This person is usually good with his hands and might gesture with them a lot. Also, this person usually likes team- building activities or group exercises.

Musical

This person is good at recognizing different rhythms, types of music, and melodies. He probably remembers melodies easily. He might have played or still be playing in a musical group. He's very likely more affected than other people by music.

Social

If you have social intelligence, you enjoy being with other people in formal and informal situations. You are adept at noticing other people's moods and listening to others. You are probably sought after by others for advice.

Environmental

Environmental intelligence is characterized with a good understanding of the natural world - plants, animals, the climate, and geography.

These people are interested in the environment and may have a concern for pets and other animals.

Practical

These people are good at sorting things out, organizing them, and putting them together coherently. They're not so much interested in theories as in seeing the theories put into practice. They're usually good at finding practical solutions to problems.

Emotional

If you have emotional intelligence, you probably are aware of and understand your own feelings and moods and how occurrences affect you. You're generally interested in self-development and may have sought counseling for your own personal self growth. You are likely to be adept at understanding other people's emotions.

Spiritual

If you have spiritual intelligence, you are concerned with fundamental questions about life. You are aware of values and principles that lie underneath actions. You may very likely be involved in community service and have a well-developed set of beliefs. You are not necessarily religious.

Chapter 4- "Successful" Intelligence

In his book, Successful Intelligence, Robert J. Sternberg offers a contemporary definition of what adds up to real, useful, sought-after intelligence. Far from the old idea of IQ, which is determined through language and math tests alone, Sternberg believes that true intelligence combines analytical, creative, and practical intelligence, resulting in real, measurable benefits and achievement of important life goals.

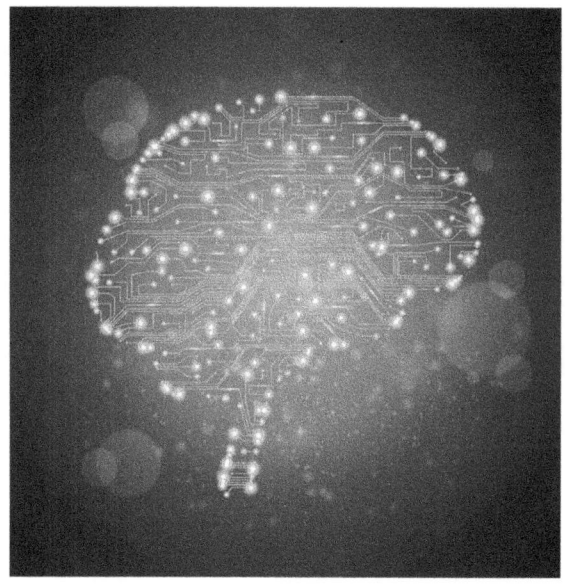

Interestingly, Sternberg, who is a Phi Beta Kappa graduate of Yale and a full professor at Yale with many grants, awards, and forty books to his name, was a "failure" in his early school years. He failed all the IQ tests in school, which he considers "lucky" because it caused him to realize at an early age that if he was going to succeed, it wouldn't be because of his IQ. He saw that people who failed IQ tests weren't necessarily unsuccessful, and people who passed them with high marks weren't necessarily successful. Sternberg began a lifelong quest to define what true intelligence is.

Sternberg claims that true intelligence is related to what really matters in life.

He says...

"People who succeed, whether by their own standards or by other people's, are those who have managed to acquire, develop, and deploy a full range of intellectual skills, rather than merely relying on the inner intelligence that schools so value. These individuals may or may not succeed on unconventional tests, but they have something in common that is much more important than high test scores. They know their strengths; they know their weaknesses. They capitalize on their strengths; they compensate for or correct their weaknesses. That's it."

Sternberg's thinking makes a lot of sense, doesn't it? There are times in life when we need to be analytical, other times when we need to be creative, and other times when we need to be practical. Furthermore, can't you think of many times when we need to be all three? This is true with small issues and with big issues alike. Have there been times when you needed to be in two places at once? You have to assess the situation, make priorities, make substitutions, and come up with the best solution possible under the circumstances.

Not only is it important to have analytical, creative, and practical abilities, but it's equally important to know when to use them.

Successful intelligence – the combination of analytical, creative, and practical intelligence – can be nurtured and developed at work, at school, and in our personal lives. Being dependent on any one

Brain Training
type of intelligence limits our full potential and the realization of our goals in life.

Chapter 5 - Styles of Learning

There are four distinct learning styles. Most people will have a preference for one of the four, but to some extent also use the others. The better you become at using all four of them, the more you will learn from your experiences. See if you can pick out the learning style that you seem to choose naturally:

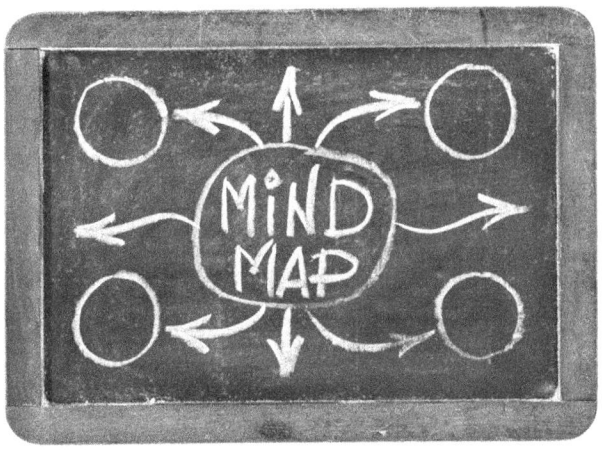

Activist Style

- This person enjoys new experiences and dives right in
- He likes the excitement of drama or a crisis
- He enjoys out-of-the-box ideas
- He likes using other people as sounding boards

Theorist Style

Brain Training

- This person enjoys theories and concepts
- She enjoys intellectual exercises
- She performs well in structured situations
- She doesn't like shallow, unsubstantial thinking

Reflector Style

- This person enjoys detailed research
- He likes just sitting back and thinking
- He thinks before he acts
- He doesn't respond well in crises or with time constraints

Pragmatist Style

- This person works well on practical tasks
- She enjoys putting things into practice immediately
- She needs guidelines
- She doesn't enjoy learning that does not have a practical outcome

Can you see that these four learning styles are all aspects of the complete learning process? At stage 1 the activist has the experience. At stage 2 the reflector reviews the experience. At stage 3 the theorist makes conclusions from the experience. And at stage 4 the pragmatist takes action based on the first three stages. Whichever style is your strong suit naturally, you can benefit from practicing all four stages.

Chapter 6- Types of Personality

One final component of brain training/thinking is your personality type. There are four types of personalities, and they determine how you approach things and how you respond to things. Remember, there is no "best" type, but understanding ourselves and others in terms of personality types can help explain why we work much better with some people than others.

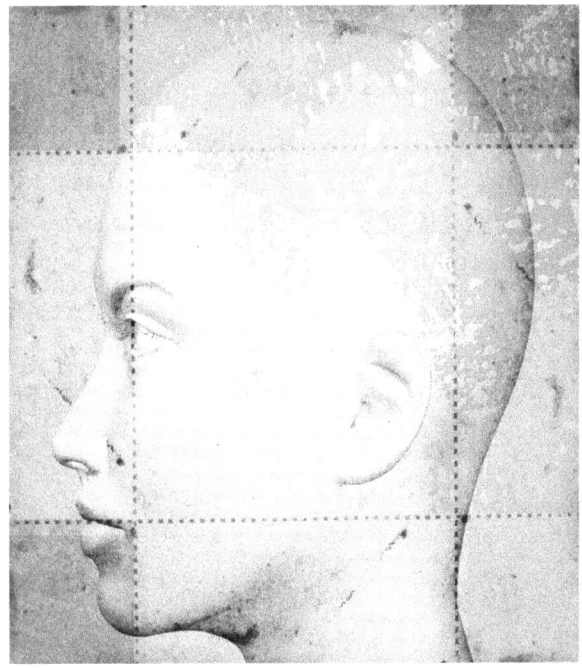

The Swiss psychiatrist, Carl Jung, was the first to investigate how our personalities affect our actions. He found that people can be divided into two groups based on how they deal with information and how they make decisions.

Sensors or Intuitors

Brain Training

These labels define how we take in and process information. Sensing people like to use their senses, while intuitive people like to use insights, associations, and connections. Neither approach is better, and even if one approach is more natural to you, you can incorporate the other one if you choose.

Thinkers and Feelers

These labels refer to how we like to make decisions. Again, neither approach is better, it's just a matter of which one you choose to do first. Thinkers certainly use feelings, and feelers certainly can think.

The benefit of understanding these labels is that you have a better understanding of how you approach information, and you have a better understanding of how other people approach information when you're working with them. This can lead to smoother sailing in your own decisions and with groups.

Chapter 7 - Self-Assessment

Now you've learned some fundamental things about the brain and how it works. You've learned that there are various types of intelligence, types of thinking, types of learning, and personality types. You've probably been able to identify which ones belong to you. As we've said before, in some categories you very likely have more than one type.

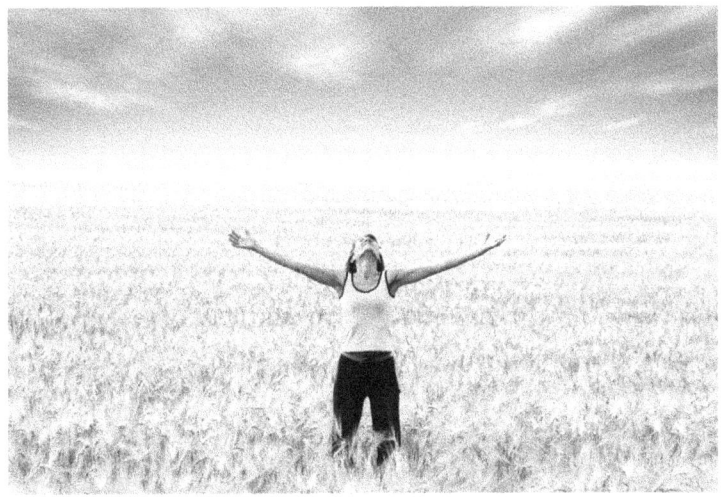

If you're having trouble deciding on your type, here are some questions to ask yourself:

1. What kind of thinker am I?
2. What's my learning style?
3. What's my personality type?
4. What blocks do I encounter in my thought process?
5. How do I go about solving problems?

6. Do I set clear goals?

7. What kind of things acts as stressors for me?

8. Which types of intelligence are my strongest?

9. Am I more an analytical thinker or a creative thinker?

10. Am I more right brain or left brain?

11. Which types of learning do I gravitate toward?

12. Which personality type am I: thinking, feeling, intuiting, or sensing?

Your first step is to establish your natural tendencies with the answers you have given to all these questions.

Then you have a choice. There are two schools of thought about maximum brain training. Both are popular, so it's up to you which way you want to go.

One, you can make a decision to strengthen your abilities by only using the thinking styles that were already prevalent in your personality. This is by far the most popular thinking currently.

Two, you can exercise your natural abilities, but also make a conscious effort to work on thinking styles that do not come so naturally to you.

The choice is really up to you, based on how you want to use your time and energy and what you think would be most beneficial for you. You might want to try each approach to see which one you like better.

CHAPTER 8- HOW TO SHARPEN

What do you think of when you think about improving your ability to "focus"?

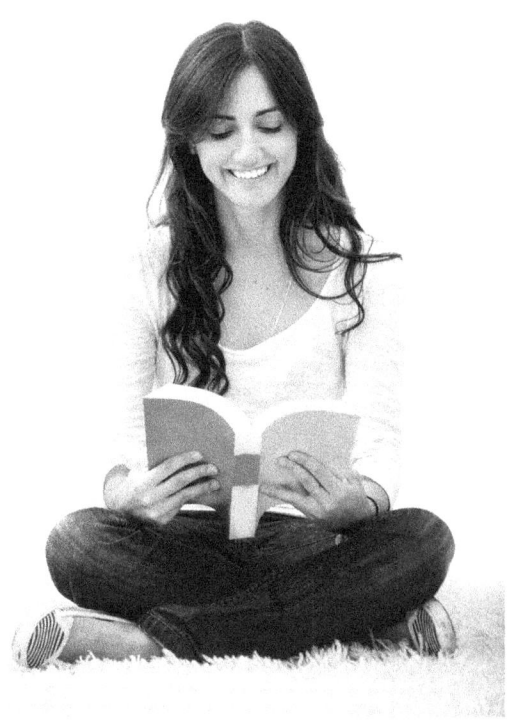

Eliminating External Distractions

There are obvious encumbrances to focus: external factors like distractions and interruptions. To remove these, you first need to recognize what they are and then exercise the self-discipline to banish them from your "space" - at least for periods of time each day.

Brain Training

These distractions can include anything from email to people stopping by. They're easy to identify, so you only need to devise a plan to deal with them and then carry it out. For some of us, saying "no" to old companions like Facebook and Skype is easier said than done, but the results are worth the effort.

Eliminating Internal Blocks

These blocks aren't so easy to identify, and there are plenty of them.

One type of block is a perceptual block. This happens when we perceive things incorrectly. For instance, when you clearly don't understand what the problem is, you can come up with ineffectual solutions or not enough solutions.

Another type of internal block is emotional. Feelings can interfere with our thinking if we let them take over. For instance, have you ever been in a meeting where you didn't understand the point that was being made, but were afraid to ask because you felt you might look foolish? How about if you're involved in something that requires taking a risk? Have you ever been convinced that making a certain move was the correct thing to do, but you didn't do it because it might not work out? Or, just the opposite, have you ever been so excited about something that you didn't think it through before taking action?

These are just some examples where emotions can get in the way of focus and clear thinking. You can probably think of many more.

Another block to clear focus is not having complete or correct information. It's very frustrating to put a lot of time and energy into a project and then realize that the conclusion will be flawed due to lack of supporting information.

It's a good idea to take a little time to sort out where you're coming from perceptually, emotionally, and practically before initiating a project.

The Habit of Successful Focus

In their excellent book, The Power of Focus, Jack Canfield, Mark Victor Hansen, and Les Hewitt discussed the idea that successful living is all about cultivating the habit of focusing on the right things. Here's what they say:

"Life doesn't just happen to be. It's all about choices and how you respond to every situation. If you are in the habit of continually making bad choices, disaster often occurs. Your everyday choices ultimately determine whether you end up living with abundance or living in poverty. Consistent choices lay the foundation for your habits. And your habits play a major role in how your future unfolds."

A habit is anything you do so often that it becomes easy. Rule of thumb is that it takes about 21 days to create a new habit. A really interesting fact is that once you do something 21 to 30 times, it's harder not to do it than to do it.

The good news is that you can begin to reprogram yourself anytime. Once you learn about yourself – how you think and feel, and what you want in life – it will be easier to make the choices that will turn into habits that fulfill your goals.

Think about that. If you only changed four habits every year, in five years you would have 20 positive new habits. Imagine how much your life would change with 20 positive habits. You can make these changes in any area you choose. It could be your health, income,

Brain Training

relationships, or any other area. 20 new habits could vastly change your overall lifestyle.

Here's something that may be news to you: your outward behavior is the truth, while your inner perception of your behavior is often an illusion. What that means is that sometimes we let ourselves off the hook and see things in a rosier light than they really are. The first thing you should do to create new, positive habits is to make a list of all habits you think are unproductive. It's important that you understand what's holding you back so that you can change it. Seeing what you need to change and really committing to changing it are the two things you need to do to change any habit.

Canfield, Hansen, and Hewitt have created an easy-to-understand, three-step process for creating new habits:

1. Clearly identify your bad or unproductive habits – be very honest when you look at your habits and think about the long-term consequences.

For instance, as a smoker, you might say," How bad can a few cigarettes a day be?" but stop to think that 10 cigarettes a day for 20 years equals 73,000 cigarettes. That's a dramatic example. Think about the difference that changing a few of your own habits will make in your life.

2. Define your new successful habit – The easiest way to change an old bad habit is to replace it with a new, good habit. Choose your new habit and picture all the benefits and rewards you will get from adopting your new habit.

3. Create a three-part action plan – For instance, if you're giving up smoking, you could read some literature on how to stop smoking, substitute another activity for smoking, and start using a nicotine patch.

Leighton K. Baines

You must identify your old habit, clearly define your habit, and take action. Start with one habit. Focus on your three action steps and put them into practice. When you're comfortable with the new habit, you can move to the next habit you want to change.

You may have heard the expression," what we concentrate on, expands." It is so true.

Brain Training

CHAPTER 9- HOW TO ENHANCE CREATIVITY

Once upon a time, creativity was thought to belong to artists and poets. It had nothing to do with the real world and certainly nothing to do with the rest of us. Creativity was something you were born with, and that was that.

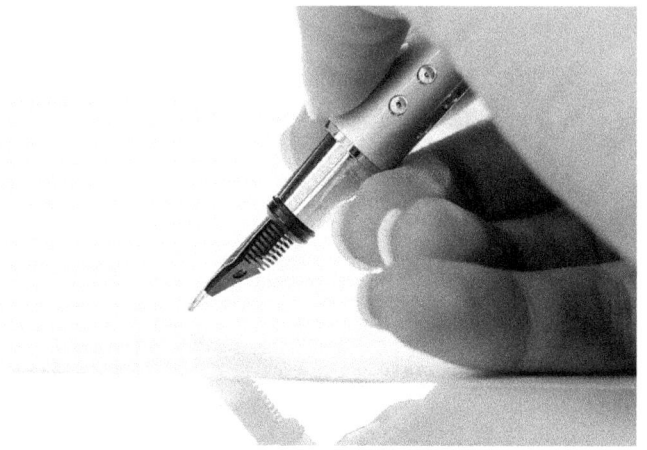

That idea has taken a 180 degree turn and bitten the dust. In our fast- moving times, whether it's in science or business or many other areas, innovation and creativity are the things that lead to success. Without them, businesses stagnate and fail.

So, what is creativity? Two French mathematicians, Hadamard and Poincarre, have defined the creative process in four steps:

1. Preparation – You discover a problem and try to solve it with established means.

2. Incubation – These methods don't work so you go off and do something else.

3. Illumination – All of a sudden, the answer appears to you.

4. Verification – You assess the new idea to see if it's any good.

It used to be thought that only two types of thinking led to creativity: convergent thinking where you draw on all your resources to solve a problem, or divergent thinking when you solve the problem by seeing it in a different way.

In the last few decades, psychologists have come to believe that there are many different ways to be creative. They think that creativity is simply a state of mind in which a person is ready and willing to entertain new ideas.

Psychologists also believe that almost all of us can learn to be more creative. Some of us may be more creative than others, but we can all be creative, especially in the areas of the 10 intelligence types, where we have our own unique strengths.

Many times we stifle our own creativity with the little voice that says," It will never work." Often we say that about other people's ideas, too. The thing you need to do is challenge that anti-creativity with a counter- argument. When you do this, you give your own creativity permission to flow.

Ask yourself open-ended questions like...

- Is there another way to do this?

- What's the worst that could happen if we tried this?

- Are there parts this idea that will work?

- What's good about this?

Brain Training
- How can we make it better?

- What can we do instead?

Practice non-judgmental idea gathering to enhance creativity.

Chapter 10 - Easy Problem Solving Techniques

When we're solving problems, enlisting a combination of some classic and new techniques will bring the best solutions.

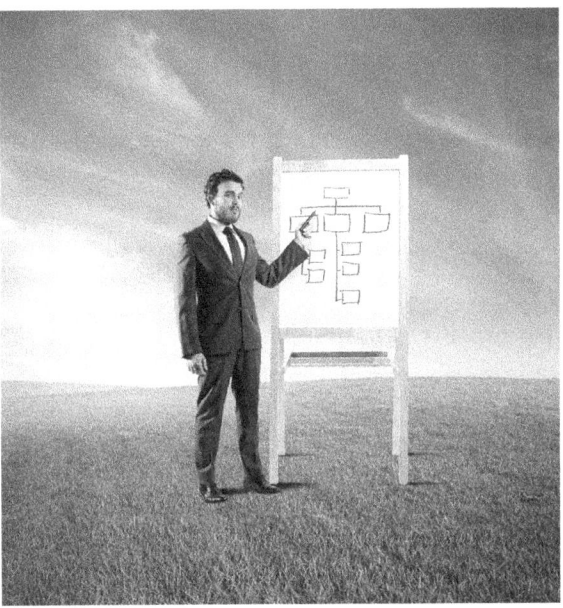

First, check your motivation. Are you bringing your best attitude to the situation? If not, try to think of the problem not is a problem, but as a challenge, a challenge that you are more than equal to finding a solution to.

Now you're ready to use the four-pronged approach for solving problems. This will give you a more well-rounded approach than if you were working with just one of your abilities.

Brain Training

1. Use your sensing abilities to look at the problem realistically, understand it, and find out what's been tried already.

2. Use your intuition to generate possibilities, go beyond present facts, and imagine future solutions.

3. Use your thinking abilities to analyze cause-and-effect relationships, prioritize, weight the criteria, and look at possible consequences of alternative solutions.

4. Use your feelings to look at the values involved and look at the human consequences of each possibility.

10 Steps to Solving a Problem

The following process is both analytical and creative. This process will work with most – not all - problems can be solved with these steps.

1. Clearly define the problem – it is not always easy, but it's absolutely necessary in order to come to the best solution.

2. Limit the problem's scope –what is the size and time of the problem? Is it for you, for other people, for a few weeks, or a few months?

3. Analyze the causes of the problem – what created this problem? What are the most likely causes? Be as complete as possible on this.

4. Write down possible solutions – at this point you're brainstorming. You want to come up with as many ideas as possible. This is non-judgmental. Don't evaluate at this point.

5. Determine your criteria for a successful solution – now that we have our ideas, we can set the criteria.

6. Refine your criteria – Not all criteria are of equal importance. Keep the ones that are critical.

7. Assess the solutions – Now we're in the analytical part of the process. Evaluate the solutions; don't throw any out too soon, but do evaluate each one thoroughly.

8. Make a decision – now that you've evaluated all the solutions, it's time to decide on the best one.

9. Take action on the solution – what's the next step in arriving at the solution to the problem? Determine the next step in the process, and take it.

10. Monitor the progress – Once the solution is up and running, evaluate how it's going.

This may seem like a lengthy process for a small project. Even so, you might want to practice this process on projects of all sizes until you become familiar with it.

Chapter 11 - Memory Improvement Techniques

Having a good memory is important, right? But have you ever stopped to consider just how important it is? The fact is that everything we do involves our memories. We can't think without using our memories, and everything that we do unconsciously, like moving our lips and making sounds to speak or walking across the street, accesses our memory, which tells us how we did it the last time.

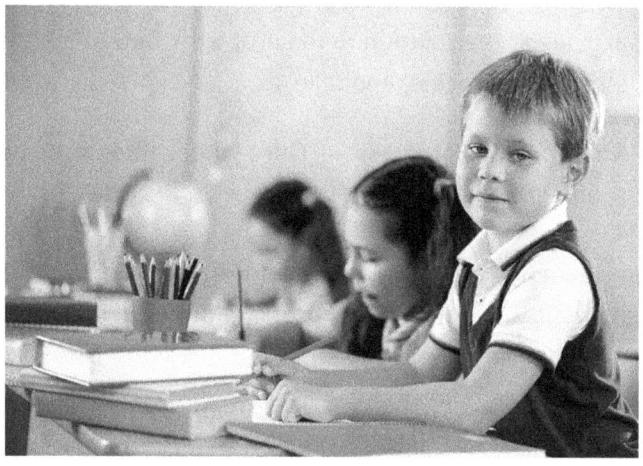

So, on one level, almost all of us have extremely good memories. These are the kinds of things we usually take for granted. We don't really think about memory at all until we find we've forgotten something. We'd like to get better at remembering things at will, and there's no reason why we can't do that since we use so little of our brains.

How Memory Works

The act of remembering something involves complex processes which utilize many parts of the brain working simultaneously. But there are only two steps involved:

- Fixing something into our memory

- Retrieving it when we need it

Here's what happens: first, we sense something (hear a statement, smell something cooking, and so on). Then an electrochemical pathway goes along neurons, across the synapses between the site of the sense and the brain. Remember, there are 10 million billion possible connections – so for our brains to remember the information accurately is an amazing feat. The more a certain pathway is activated, the better chance that memory will be created.

We have two types of memory – explicit and implicit.

Implicit memory (often-used pathways) allows us to do things automatically because those are so familiar since we've done them time after time.

Explicit memory involves things we have to remember consciously. As an example, you remember how to use the telephone automatically, but you need to consciously recall the telephone number you want to use.

We can't improve our implicit memory with exercises, but you might want to try some of these techniques to improve your explicit memory.

Motivation

Brain Training

Believe it or not, how much you want to or need to remember something plays a vital part in remembering it. If you commit yourself to remember something and concentrate on it, your chances of remembering it are much better.

Learning Process

Here's another surprising fact: studies have shown that short bursts of activity help you remember something better and for longer. Many of us got through college pulling all-nighters, so we know they work. It's true, they work better for remembering things short-term, like when you want to pass an exam. But working in short bursts of time helps us to remember things better over longer periods of time.

So if you have something that you want to remember for a long time, don't study for hours on end, but make a plan to study a part of the entire project, take a break, and go back to studying.

Physiological Alertness

Studies have shown that we do not retain things when we are at low levels of alertness, such as in sleep, or at very high levels of alertness, such as in panic or high stress. Our optimal level of alertness for learning and remembering is somewhere in between these two extremes.

Determine your own optimum alert state and save that time for learning things that are most important to you. Other things can be done when you're less alert. This approach will give you the best chance of storing information in your long-term memory.

Time of Day

Again, studies might surprise you. It had been previously thought that the best time for learning was in the morning. Studies are showing now that learning in the morning hours is better for short-term memory.

Learning later in the day seems to be better for long-term memory.

Remembering Names

Here's an area where a lot of people are self-conscious. It's embarrassing not to be able to remember someone's name, especially when that person seems to have no trouble remembering yours. This is like every other aspect of memory – some people are at a higher level of unconscious competence in this area, and they remember names by using a process even if they don't know it. If you make a conscious decision to remember someone's name and follow these steps, you too will be successful in remembering names in the future.

1. Consciously decide to give this person respect by learning his name

2. Listen when you hear the name. It's easy to be focusing on other things and let the name slip by.

3. Be certain that you hear his name properly. If there's any doubt, ask him to spell it.

4. Visualize that you've written the name down. Doing this forces you to listen to it. This visualization is a surprisingly powerful technique.

5. Visualize the name itself. Seeing the name in your mind acts as a trigger. If you can associate it with something else like a town or a famous person, it becomes even stronger.

Brain Training

> Associate the person in front of you who belongs to the name with the name in your mind, so that the name and the person's face are linked in your mind.

Triggers for Stubborn Memories

You can probably relate to this – sometimes we have problems remembering things even though we very much want to remember them. Criminal investigations use techniques that can help us with recalling our own memories. Here's what you do:

1. Recreate the original conditions in your mind. See them as clearly as possible and use your senses. What was happening? How did you feel? Was it hot or cold? Were you tired, hungry, angry, at the time?

2. Pay attention to the details, even the unimportant ones. What do you see? Those images may help you bring other images to mind.

3. Try to see the situation from another point of view. For instance, if you were sitting in a chair the last time you saw your ring, pretend you're standing in the doorway looking at the situation. What you see now?

4. See the situation in reverse. In your mind, see the situation before you entered it. See the room before you came into it – what was happening then?

5. These "investigation" techniques are powerful for recalling stubborn memories.

It's Just Physical

Studies show that the relationship between physical fitness and mental ability is powerful. Exercise can boost mental capacity by about 25%. In addition to physical activity, you should pay some attention to your hearing and eyesight. All of these factors play a part in how well you think and how well you remember things.

Finally, take a minute to think about any medication you're on. Of course, physical conditions absolutely do need drugs sometimes. Don't take any action to change drug dosages without consulting your physician, but drugs can seriously affect your ability to think and to remember.

Brain Training

CHAPTER 12- AUTOTELIC THINKING

There are exercises that can help you think better, faster, more clearly. I hope you've found some of them in this book so far.

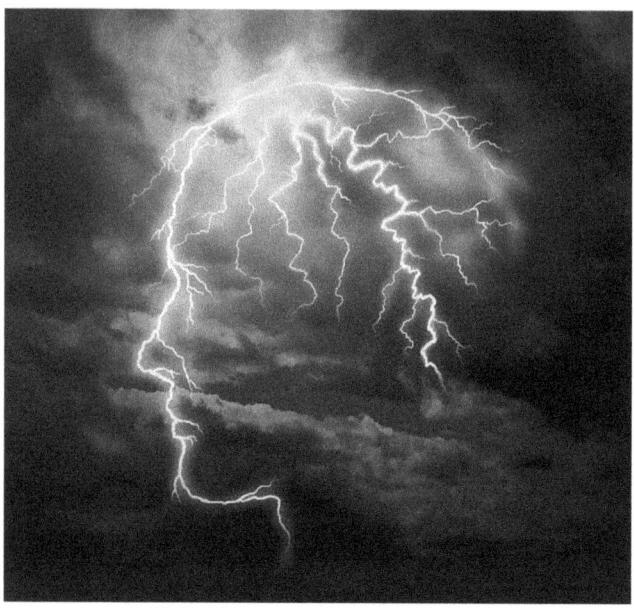

And then there are insights that can change your life. Autoletic thinking turns problems into challenges to be met and learned from. It is an approach that will change your life if you practice it.

Mihaly Csikszentmihalyi is the author of Flow: The Psychology of Optimal Experience, a remarkable book in which he discusses how our thinking can enhance our quality of life. He explains how a rich, strong, powerful person is no more in control of his consciousness than someone who is sickly, poor, weak, or oppressed. The difference is whether he sees challenges as threats or as opportunities for action.

Leighton K. Baines

What he calls the autotelic self refers to someone who has the ability to translate potential threats into enjoyable challenges, and thus has an internal balance. The term autotelic self means a person who has self-contained goals. For most people, goals are shaped by biological needs and social conventions – things which are outside the self. The difference is that the autotelic self, or the person who is capable of defining things for himself, is also capable of transforming threats into non-threatening challenges. This can be done with a simple change of perspective, a shift in consciousness: that is, seeing a threat as a challenge that you can overcome. Once you can do that, the steps are simple:

1. Be crystal clear about the goal. Once you know exactly what the goal is, you have an understanding of what is needed to meet it. Then you can decide on a series of actions necessary to accomplish the goal. You can modify these actions as needed in order to meet the goal.

2. Become involved in the activity -- This means commitment. This means action. Whether things are going your way or not, you consistently take action with the next best steps. This demands concentration, commitment, and follow through.

3. Pay attention to what is happening – This really means that the project becomes more important than your own feelings about what is happening. Your concentration is on the results of the project. You invest your energy in the project. You are committed, you are involved – it's about the project, not about you.

4. Enjoying the experience – the autotelic self is able to set goals, develop skills, be sensitive to feedback, get involved, and look past obstacles. The benefit of learning to be an

autotelic personality is that anything that happens can be a source of joy because it is a source of learning and step to the next goal. In other words, there are no failures, only learning experiences.

This approach to thinking can mean the difference between living life in fear or living life in joy. Developing autotelic thinking will give you the ability to transform random events into learning experiences that eventually result in success. Life is change - by definition and for everyone. Seeing that as a challenge to be accepted, enjoyed, and built on is the "secret" to successful living.

Leighton K. Baines

Chapter 13- Maintaining Brain Power

We've all heard about the mind-body connection, and as we saw in the chapter on memory, it's real. What that means is that peak performance mentally requires a healthy body, emotional well-being, and a balanced lifestyle.

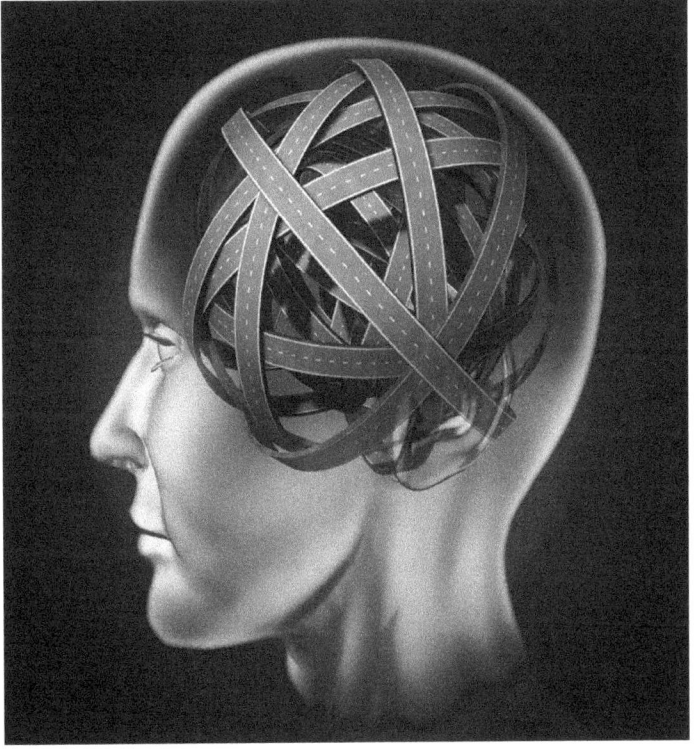

We'll discuss a few key points here. You can find more detailed information about the subjects in many other places. Here are some highlights.

Healthy Living

Brain Training

Drinking water – believe it or not, most of us live in a constant state of partial dehydration. This means that our brain functions at less than full capacity. Alcohol dehydrates us and reduces the flow of blood to our brains, which reduces our thinking power. Caffeine does increase our alertness in the short term, but also dehydrates us.

The rule is that you should drink eight glasses of water a day and two glasses of water for every cup of coffee you drink.

Eating smart – most of us already know the rules about eating healthy. Unfortunately, it's easier and tastier to eat things that are not good for us. Anyway, a healthy diet consists of the right amounts of protein, complex carbohydrates, and good fats. That means avoiding a lot of things we like, such as processed foods, fried foods, desserts full of simple sugars, and high-fat foods. Instead, concentrate on eating protein, fruits and vegetables, complex carbs, and drinking less water.

Grazing, eating small meals (about 250 to 350 calories a meal) instead of eating three big meals a day, is finding great favor with nutritionists currently because it helps to maintain level blood sugar. It also helps maintain a more constant state of mental alertness, energy, and performance throughout the day.

Sleep – everyone needs to process what happened during each day, and that's done during periods of deep sleep. Exactly how many hours of sleep you need each night is an individual thing that you should determine for yourself, but over time, lack of sleep can lead to poor concentration, low energy, mood swings, and even poor mental health.

Fun/enjoyment – we all need it, even workaholics. Research shows us that taking part in some activities that we enjoy reduces our stress level and improves our immune system.

Leighton K. Baines
Brain Training – Like most things, it's in your hands. You now have many scientifically proven and currently popular techniques that will work for you if you use them. Best wishes for your great success!

Chapter 14 - What Is Manifestation?

Every individual has reasons why he or she wants to manifest what they like for his or her own life.

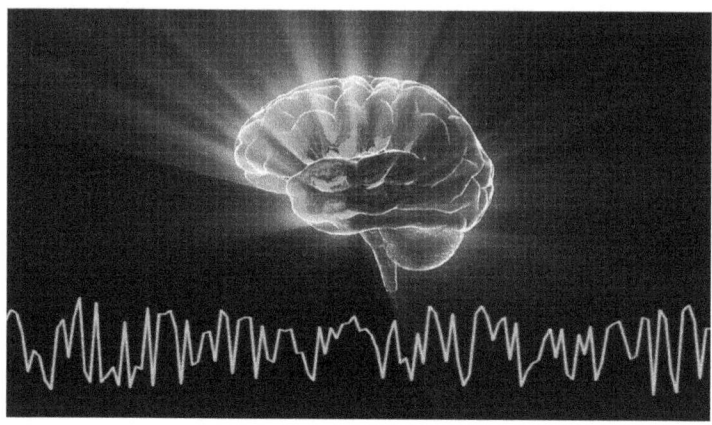

The Basics

But, how can you master the art of manifestation? What are the things that you need to consider? Why do you need to manifest something?

There are different approaches that you may take in consideration when making manifestations. These approaches may vary depending on how the person handles the situation.

But, before everything else, you have to know what manifestation means before you take any necessary steps. You also have to know the abilities required for you to make successful manifestation. This is because there are things that may assist you while you are applying the steps to manifest anything.

So, what are really the secrets to successful manifestation and why do you need to master it? Is it a requirement in this life?

Or, is it another way for you to be successful in life? The answer is simple and it depends on the person.

For those who are not familiar with manifestation, it is best described as co-creating your dreams by facing reality and accepting everything. It is also getting rid of negatives while you are on your journey.

What's the Fuss?

These negatives may be anything that holds you back while trying to manifest something that you desire. But, most of the common negatives are fear and lack of patience. That is the reason why some don't have the guts to face the changes and don't like to take risks, as they are afraid to lose something that they may not afford to lose.

Many individuals have higher levels of fear rather than faith. It is true that it is in the nature of every human being, but you can do something to get rid of it and that is by embracing them and applying solutions slowly. Rushing things won't give you great results. It may provide you a quick solution, but it will never resolve everything.

There are various tips that you may consider when you want to perfect successful manifestation. First and foremost, you need to be patient. You will obtain success in the right time and the right place.

Brain Training

You can't rush it unless you have a time machine that will let you enter your future world. Second, clear your state of mind and focus on your goals.

If you can't concentrate on your goals, you will always be confused and will face tough times. Clearing your mind involves eliminating negative emotions and letting positive vibes rule.

When clearing your mind, you also need to get out of your shell and view the beauty of the world. This will keep you energized and will give you strength to face your journey. With a clear and positive mind, you'll have the power to manifest anything. All you need to do is believe that you can do it.

Chapter 15- Why People Have Problems Manifesting

Many people don't seem to manifest effectively because they let their negative attitudes reign. They fear facing reality and don't want to take the challenge because they think that it would be risky for them to face the truth and go with the flow of reality.

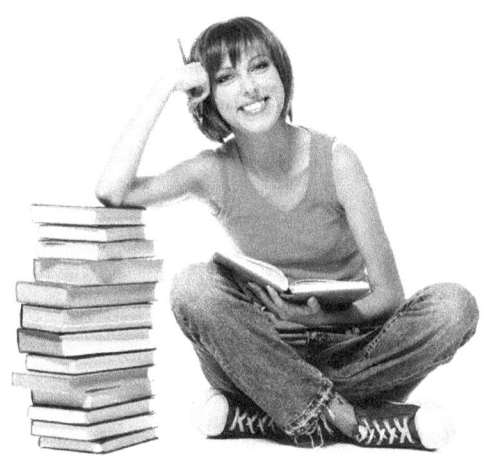

Also, they think that reality sucks and their life would be much easier if they ignore reality. Since not all people are the same, they have different approaches to every situation. Some manifest by playing it safe while others manifest without knowing the behind the scene facts of the situation.

This is because some are open-minded about the situation while others just concentrate for their own good and they want to make sure that they will get success in life.

What Happens

Brain Training

Manifesting or co-creating your dreams or wants in life is not easy for everyone. It is a crucial process with various steps and it may take some time for others to master it. Apart from fears, there are other reasons why some people don't seem to manifest successfully.

One of these reasons is that many don't want to accept the change. There are a number of individuals that don't want to take a step to accept the change because they think that it would be just a waste of time and they have a high level of belief in their old ways.

Some even don't like to experience change as this could just ruin their overall plan and feel it is just useless if they take any steps to embrace change.

But, what others really don't know is that manifesting is about accepting the reality and letting go of their negative attitudes that keep them from manifesting. If you are one of the persons that have these negative things in life, you will never succeed in manifesting.

So, if you want to achieve your dreams in life and want to be successful with your business or personal life, then taking away such negative factors in your life could be your first step.

Once you have done this successfully, you will never have those tough times and it will be a lot easier for you to proceed to the next level of manifestation.

If you have experienced any hard times while you are in the process, don't give up and keep improving your courage because once you pay attention to the bad things, you will not be effective in manifesting and will keep failing. If this happens, just remember your goals, why you're doing it and keep the positive vibes so you can master manifestation without encountering tough times.

Chapter 16- Presumptions about Manifestation

Manifestation is about doing your best to attain your goals and facing the reality without any hesitations. It is not about expecting the outcome of your decision.

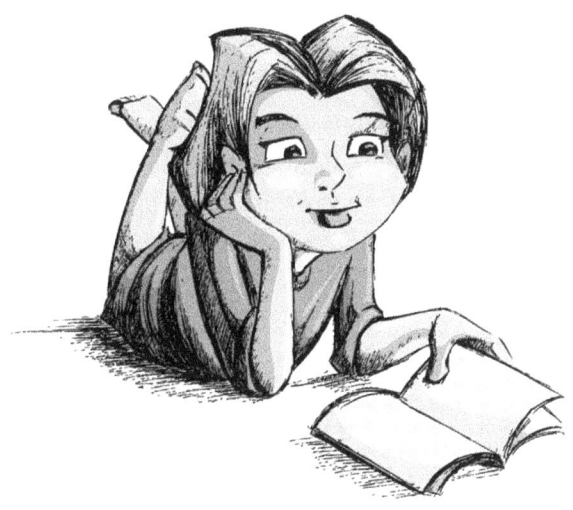

Of course, many people wait for different things that may come after taking a step because they are afraid to fail. But, if you will just keep on assuming and not doing anything, you won't reach your goals in life.

To get successful manifestation, the first thing that you should do is to empty your preconceptions. Do not formulate things in your

Brain Training

mind as you can't do it or you don't have the power to achieve what you want.

Preconceptions about manifestation are like not trying to fix the things that hinder you from making your vision into reality.

Examine It Well

If you keep preconceptions, you won't succeed at anything and stay in the same place where you are right now. If your life is a vehicle, you will always get stuck in traffic and it would take you too long to get to your destination.

Preconceptions are sometimes good because they let you imagine the possibilities. But, oftentimes, they are the negative elements that you must get rid of because if they pollute your mind, you won't be able to get successful manifestation.

You can empty preconceptions about manifestation by starting to embrace the good things that it may give you. Always stay positive and think of your rewards once you have achieved your desires. This will keep your spirit up and you will be energized all the time. It is okay to have preconceptions about manifestation, but if you will not get rid of it, then, you won't get the concept of manifestation successfully. Another step that you may consider when getting rid of preconceptions is by knowing the essential things for consideration.

Also, don't forget the things that you should be aware of because they can be a great help in the future. Once you have rid yourself of preconceptions about manifestation, you will never get lost on your path to development and you will reach your dreams in no time.

Chapter 17 - Setting Your Intention - The Importance of It

For every action you take, you should know your intention and why you want to do it because if you don't know your goals, you won't be able to stay on the path and you will keep on failing in getting what you want. Take note, it is hard to manifest anything that you imagine. So, for you to do it successfully, you have to set your intention before anything else.

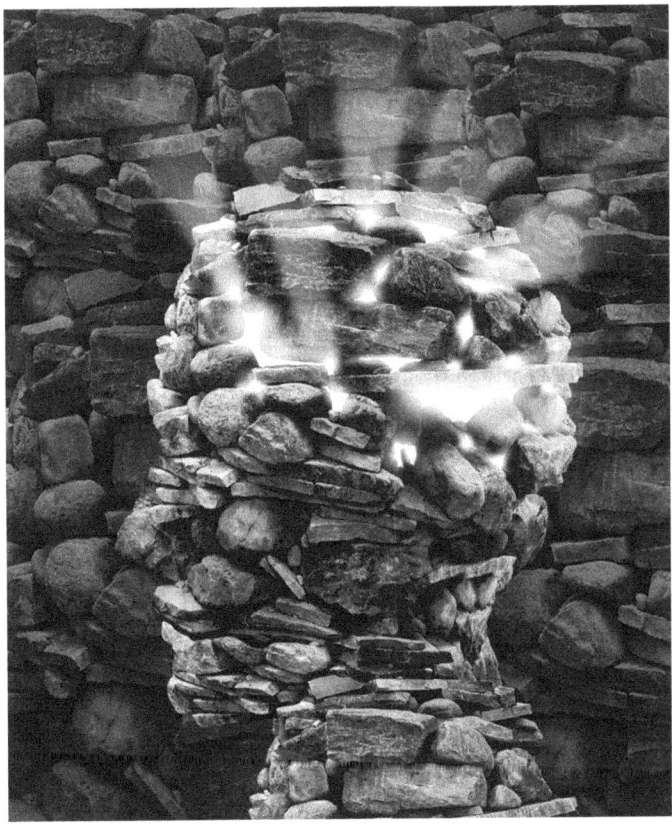

Getting It Together

Brain Training

Setting your intention is very important because this could serve as your guide or note that would remind you what you really want for your life. If you don't know your intention, start by determining your goals and the things you want to achieve in your personal or business life. If you have goals in mind, try to write it down and keep the list with you. You may aim for anything as long as it would make your life much better.

Your intentions will also determine the things that you need for you to stay on the path to successful manifestation. If you are still confused about your intentions, try to take everything slow and don't rush setting your intentions. The reason behind it is that you may concentrate on one thing and forgot to include the things that you may need while you are in the process. You also have to bear in mind that it can be complex to consider all the things you want. It is because this may just confuse you and might not give you the positive results that you want to get.

When setting your intentions, only include the vital things that would benefit you. If you think that one of your goals may just ruin what you want to achieve, then, remove it. Don't set your intentions individually because it would not lead you to the results that you wanted to achieve. If possible, concentrate only on what you really want and eliminate the things that may not give you any rewards.

Importance Faith When Manifesting

Faith will serve as your energy when you want to manifest something. Without this, you will never make it to the top and won't get what you desire. Unfortunately, only a few have a huge amount of energy levels in their bodies because they always let negative things invade their minds.

You likely have relied on faith if you have gone through difficulties in the past few years. But, if this is your first time to manifest anything, you might find it difficult to gain high levels of faith.

Everybody needs to have faith in himself or herself. However, some don't know how to use this at times that they are experiencing tough times because they react to the situation. There are tons of reasons why some people can't manage their faith. One of these reasons is that they thought when they kept on being positive and believing that everything would turn out fine, it would just get worse.

Faith

Some say that it is a talent to keep your faith because almost everyone is easily influenced by temptations and think negatively. Based from a reliable source, experts said that people are quickly tempted because they think that such things will change the situation and everything will be solved.

Getting tempted is part of one's life. But, you should learn how to avoid temptations and maximize your faith as this thing could take you anywhere and would keep you moving forward.

Having faith is like having a powerful tool that you could use whenever there are challenges that tear you down.

With your faith, the term impossible will never be in your vocabulary and you won't get depressed with the outcome because you believe that you will get it right next time.

Most of you know how hard it is to manifest what you really want, but if you will keep the faith, you will charge yourself with good

Brain Training

energy and everything you want in life will be in your hands in no time.

But, how can you improve your faith? It is not simple to improve faith. But, it is possible for you to do it. Some take necessary steps to improve their faith. Improving faith does not suggest that you need to be religious and become a holy man.

All you need is to believe that you will get what you want. Others misinterpret the concept of improving faith because they think that having faith means becoming a religious individual. Well, it may be, but it depends on the. So, the ways may depend on what you believe in.

Whether you want to reach your goals or make money effectively, making manifestation a permanent habit is essential. It may be hard for some people to do it, but if you know the dos and dont's about manifestation and you know how to unblock yourself from the said blockages, you will manifest effectively.

Co-creating things that you want to take time and sometimes, you need to undergo a crucial process before you learn everything about the law of attraction and art of manifestation.

For you to stay on the right path, you need to adapt all the lessons you have learned in life and be open to whatever may come. Preparedness is also another important thing that you should not forget. Be prepared all the time because challenges may strike you anytime to test your emotional capabilities and strength to face such problems.

Also, do not expect too much about the outcome because you might get the opposite result of the stuff that you need to do for you to get the secret of successful manifestation. If the world offers you challenges, embrace them and try to seek some ways that would help you get rid of them. And, do not make failure your habit. Instead, make manifestation your permanent habit and improve your lifestyle.

Don't think that you can't make manifestation a permanent habit because everything can be done easily as long as you have faith and will to do it. Thus, get what you want in life and live in a better way.

ABOUT THE AUTHOR

Leighton K. Baines is a man who likes adventure and loves to find out more information on what the mind can do. It is something that is fascinating to him as the true power of the mind is yet to be truly discovered by scientists. He does his own research and has found quite a number of schools of thought to be plausible.

What he presents in his book is a look at the brain, how it really works and how persons can unlock that hidden potential that we hear spoken about so often.

www.ingramcontent.com/pod-product-compliance
Ingram Content Group UK Ltd.
Pitfield, Milton Keynes, MK11 3LW, UK
UKHW022219230426
12048UKWH00016BA/939